THE NURSING HOME DILEMMA

BY: URSULA A. FALK AND GERHARD FALK

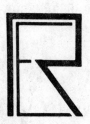

San Francisco, California
1976

Published in 1976 by

R AND E RESEARCH ASSOCIATES
4843 Mission Street, San Francisco 94112
18581 McFarland Avenue, Saratoga, California 95070

Publishers and Distributors of Ethnic Studies
Adam S. Eterovich
Robert D. Reed

Library of Congress Card Catalog Number
75-36565

ISBN
0-88247-399-9

INTRODUCTION

The present study describes in some detail what an aged American may expect if he enters a nursing home.

It is our view that the treatment of the old in both public and private nursing homes is the outgrowth of the view of old age generally held in America and other industrial countries and that the self image of the aged therefore contributes to the treatment received.

We have shown in a brief first chapter that the treatment of the old is but a reflection of a general view of mankind as developed in our civilization. We have then illustrated this thesis in a number of case histories of patients now living in nursing homes or dying there. The reader should view these case histories, selected from a much larger group known to us, as typical. This may be hard to do, as these cases will seem extreme to the uninitiated. We contend that they are common and expected.

We have discussed several critical issues in the treatment of aged nursing home patients and followed this with a statistical study of staff attitudes concerning such patients.

It is our opinion that staff attitudes as here described support the case history material cited earlier and are again a reflection of the general view of aging in America.

We have made numerous suggestions for improving the lot of the aged nursing home patient but are also convinced that true improvement can only come when we remember the admonition of Leviticus (Lev. XIX 32), "Thou shalt rise before the hoary head and honor the face of the old."

INDEX

PART I

Old Age in America

"...the aged are mistreated, even in the best of nursing homes."[1]
With this statement the author of one of the most significant works on
the treatment of the aged in American society summarizes the "Nursing
Home Dilemma." For the essence of that dilemma is this: while the number of Americans over 65 now makes up one tenth of the population[2], i.e.,
a number equal to all blacks in America or equal to the entire population
of California, this group of over 20 million Americans is also the most
marginal of our people for American society shuns its elders and imperils
its humanity by relegating this vast group to living facilities which
reduce the "life space" of the "senior citizen" to an institutionalized
routine which is diametrically opposed to all these values which Americans and technological men everywhere hold so dear[3]. Such values are
generally derived from urban attitudes but are also founded on older
American experiences as embodied in that state of mind principally asso-
ciated with Calvinism. Thus, these values of independence, self suffi-
ciency and the right to make individual choices are tremendously important
to anyone who has lived his life in America. Yet, nursing home care ipso
facto deprives the patient of all these opportunities. Therefore, the
mistreatment of the aged in nursing homes need not be deliberate or con-
scious mistreatment by the staff but can arise out of the dilemma here

indicated. The question we must ask in this connection is: how can we be independent when our agility is impaired by old age and we cannot climb the steps into a bus, let alone run after one? How can we be independent when old age robs us of our vision and we cannot get about in a city which hardly has public transportation even if we could walk to the street corner from our house? If shopping facilities are principally developed in suburbs where younger people live and where large shopping centers keep prices down, while small stores in deteriorated areas where older people live cost more, then the old, who are generally poor, must pay more[4]. Thus, paradoxically, it is in the most deteriorated areas of the big American cities that most aged Americans must live. Even the redevelopment of such areas does the old and poor no good. For when an area has been redeveloped, rents rise and the aged cannot pay them. When new shopping facilities are installed, the whole area becomes more efficient, less personal, and very much dependent on the customers' mobility. All this is directly contrary to the competence, both physical and financial, of the aged. Therefore it would appear that institutionalization is the answer as such a move appears to provide all those services which lack of physical stamina, lack of money and failing agility will no longer allow.

2

We have already seen that the difficulties of being old in America are derived from a life style which is predicated on the assumption that everyone is young and able bodied. Yet, the age of the American population is rising, so that there were nearly eight million Americans over 75 in 1973[5].

Therefore, the presence of the aged cannot be denied or "swept under the rug." Something must be done to secure the lives of all these people and something has been done. That "something" is called "Medicare" and consists of a Federal government subsidy, automatically offering hospitalization benefits to anyone whose age can be verified by a Social Security card. However, these "benefits" seldom improve the condition of the institutionalized aged. Instead, the chief beneficiaries of "Medicare" are professionals and institutions who collect as much as $13 billion a year from this plan, so that some physicians earn as much as $25,000 from these plans alone[6]. Since money is made primarily by institutionalizing as many people as possible, a large number of the aged are placed into "nursing" home facilities when in fact they do not necessarily or permanently need such care. In fact, two-thirds of patients in the 65 to 69 age group and one-half of patients in the 70 to 79 age group were inappropriately placed. This error in placement was almost exclusively in the direction of excessive and unnecessary institutionalization[7]. However, "half way" houses are seldom available, since such facilities do not provide private operators with the profits that so-called medical and health related facilities will provide. This does not mean that "nursing homes" necessarily have medical care or even one nurse on duty. It only means that the operators of such places make such claims. It is for this reason that 225 "nursing homes" were decertified by HEW in 1969 as that agency discovered then that these homes did not meet their minimum standards, i.e., the presence of one nurse on duty during one eight hour shift per day[8]. There are, of course, a few extremely expensive, well run and efficient nursing homes. However, the efforts by HEW to use Medicare to improve all the others must fail because of the profit motive. Thus, as more money is paid by government for nursing home care, the care does not improve. Instead, the costs for the same poor care go up. In addition, more and more nursing homes are built and developed so that businessmen can share in the profits. This in turn leads to an ever larger number of spaces whence children can "dump" their elders in order to rid themselves of those whose mere presence annoys them in a "gerontophobic" society[9].

Essentially then, the existence of nursing homes, whether good, bad or indifferent, is the result of values in America and has to do with the view we take of age, much more than with the profit motive, although that too is so heavily involved. An excellent example of the tremendous power of the profit motive was the 1972 amendment of the Social Security Act[10], which rescinded the 1966 provision that any nursing home wishing government licensing or reimbursement must have a social worker on its staff. However, "hiring professional social workers increases operating expenses and reduces profits"[11] and was therefore eliminated by Congress.

We thus have a society which views men as objects or merchandise and makes so-called nursing homes nothing more than store houses for those whose economic functions are impaired. This means that the earning power of the old has been reduced or totally eliminated because they cannot work or are not permitted to work. In fact, work is so important a portion of the lives of Americans that most find it difficult to accept retirement. Even persons in their fifties and sixties, younger than 65, find it hard to discover employment opportunities, particularly since an ever increasing

4

pool of unemployed younger workers resent older applicants while employers view them as irritants[12]. However, the old become economically important again because they represent the raw material stored in warehouses called "nursing homes." The concept here is exactly the same as that enunciated by Adolf Eichman at his trial in Jerusalem where he told the court in 1961 that he had no hatred of the Jews he murdered but merely viewed them as "Ware" (pron. Vaare), the German word for "wares."[13]

The treatment of the old as merchandise is of course related to the treatment Americans give one another long before old age insures the final rejection. This treatment is largely based on economic position, but is primarily related to occupation. "In contemporary America", says Slocum, "the type of work a man does must be regarded as among the principal determinants of his social rank."[14] In fact, occupation is used by sociologists as the principal indicator of prestige and social class, a judgment well founded upon numerous opinion polls. Most important of these polls were those made by the National Opinion Research Center in 1947 and again in 1963 which plainly showed that occupations having not only a good income but a high degree of responsibility, independence and self determination ranked the highest among the 90 occupations evaluated[15]. This then leads us to the inescapable conclusion that those who are retired, and particularly those who are institutionalized, share none of the admired characteristics, but on the contrary exhibit the opposite attitudes. They appear dependent, not responsible for their own lives, and surely lack all self determination. Thus their prestige is the lowest and their treatment resembles their prestige. Therefore, old age begins in childhood, in America as elsewhere, for the outcome of youth must be age. Consequently, it is inevitable that a society which rewards the one must punish the other. This punishment consists of institutionalization, a means which guarantees that the old patient, or anyone institutionalized, will lose those prerequisites for independence which are the essential requirement of American self esteem.

In an excellent discussion of children's rights, Mergers has shown diagrammatically how institutions reduce the range of choices as the rigidity of the structures increases. His diagram is well worth reproducing here since it applies to nursing homes as well. It should be borne in mind, however, that this reduction in available choices is ordinarily only temporary for the child and the middle aged hospital patient while for the old it is permanent, relieved only by death.

Chart 1.[16]

ORGANIZATIONAL COMPLEXITY STRUCTURE

Choices	Structural Rigidity
100%	100% of options predetermined by structural requirements
Options	Percent of available for individual choice
0%	Independent living

The case of Romera Black illustrates adequately the fate of many a nursing home patient. It is not exaggerated but common and repeatable a million times.

Case 1 - ROMERA BLACK

Mrs. Romera Black had lived a peaceful existence with her husband until he died suddenly of a heart attack. Mrs. Black had a very difficult time coping with her loneliness. She had no close relatives and her friends had passed away one after the other until she remained in her large apartment with only an occasional telephone call. She approached a distant cousin for advice and because she felt she could not live "all alone" he urged her to enter a nursing home "for a while." Being in a vulnerable position she very mildly and without much discussion consented to do so. Her cousin had promised to look for some help for her after she was placed and he could find some help in a leisurely fashion.

In the beginning Mrs. B. almost welcomed the regimentation of the Home. She knew she had to be in the dining room for breakfast by eight, that she would be asked to take her bath next, and that then she could go back into her room where her roommate rocked and talked a bit. Then came lunch, etc. Her depression over her loss was great and she was not extremely interested in her surroundings. She would do the bidding of the aides quietly and without outward emotion. Her gait became slower and assumed a shuffling motion as time went on and this rather soft spoken woman became almost totally silent. She would answer questions asked of her in a bland affectless fashion but would not initiate conversation. The attendants would call her "cute" and put bright bows in her hair to "perk her up." Mrs. B. just smiled her sterile meaningless smile which appeared grotesque in her masklike face.

7

Her cousin visited her twice during the first year of her stay at Haven Manor but then stopped altogether. It was obvious that he had little interest in her - for she could do nothing for him - and he no longer considered her among the living.

After two years of routinized existence, Mrs. B. suffered from a prolapsed rectum. She cried out in agony and eventually was transferred by ambulance to a local hospital and soon returned to the Haven since "nothing much could be done for her." She had become a welfare patient and little money could be made on extensive medical care for this very thin, depressed white haired lady. Mrs. B.'s screams from the pain became so pronounced that she was removed to a small dark room called the "tub" room - a unit removed some distance from the staff and the other inmates. Despite this her cries and screams were audible and she could be heard: "God give me meat, God give me bread, God give me love." In her helplessness she could no longer appeal to people who had treated her in an inhumane fashion. The attendants became so annoyed that at first they closed the door to her room. When the State examiners were coming to the Haven to investigate the nursing home, a verbal order was issued by the Administrator to the head nurse to the RN that the patient was to receive strong dosages of tranquilizers. When the first dosage did not achieve the required result and Mrs. B. screamed louder, adding "God give me peace" to her recitation, the nurse following orders from the aforementioned authorities repeated the dosage in a lethal form. When the examiners walked into Mrs. B.'s room she appeared to be asleep but was actually in a coma; when they had gone Romera suffered no more - all cries for help were stilled within her forever. She was dead!

PART II

The Silent Ones, the Good Ones

The nursing home is a mirror image of American society. Whereas independence, self determination and "rugged individualism" are at least given "lip service," the opposite is true in the nursing home. The "Silent Ones, the Good Ones" are the object of the nursing home employees' affection; and this every patient who wants to be a "success" must learn. Who are the "good patients?"

Let us introduce you to some nursing home "successes:"

Case 2 - Paul Fenster

Mr. Paul Fenster was a genteel looking gentleman with a shock of thick white hair, blue eyes that always looked a little misty and a sad smile. Paul had a severe limp as the result of a railroad accident which had caused permanent damage to his hip socket and which made every step a painful one. He was completely toothless, but the nursing home in which he lived refused to send someone with him for a denture fitting. Mr. Fenster had saved $500 from his meager $24.50 a month allowance and could well afford the much needed appliances. When he requested "teeth" he was shunted aside with "when someone has time; do you think we are here only just for you?" and with that Mr. Fenster would retreat into his room leaning heavily on his cane. Occasionally he would wipe the tears from his cloudy blue eyes.

9

When the social worker approached the nursing home administrator with Paul's problem she was told that he "is just a dirty old man" and should have taken care of his teeth before he arrived at Haven Manor.

Mr. Fenster had come to the nursing home two years earlier after a long hospitalization for his hip injury. He had lived alone in a room prior to this, since he had no relatives who were interested in him. His wife had died in a mental hospital many years ago and their daughter had moved south without leaving a forwarding address; one son who lived in a room in Buffalo refused to deal with his father, claiming that he had his own problems and did not feel like traveling the distance to Haven Manor. Thus Mr. Fenster was left to the mercy of strangers, namely, Haven Manor's staff.

Mr. Fenster had a hearing problem in addition to his many other physical anomalies. He could not remember names because he could not hear them. He would call the staff by the color of their hair, i.e., "Blackie," "Blondie," etc. He would also describe the patients with whom he had any sort of relationship by their physical debilities, i.e., the lady with the double cane, or the man with the skull cap. He was paired off at the table with a temperamental young invalid who would often have extreme mood swings. On one of those occasions Mr. Fenster's table partner threw a cup of coffee in his face, burning his cheeks and soiling his trousers.

Mr. Fenster was almost devoid of clothes as well as of other material possessions. His trousers were held together by safety pins which would occasionally open and be a source of great annoyance to him. Instead of helping him, the staff were very judgmental and attributed his condition to "his own fault."

His only source of joy was a harmonica which a sister once had given him during her Christmas visit to him. He loved to play that instrument and played it well. One day when the nursing home administrator came out of her office (a rare occurrence since she did not like to mingle with patients) she heard music coming from the chapel where Paul played his harmonica. The "Marm" (administrator) became so annoyed that she walked into the chapel, screamed at the old man and told him never to play "that piece of junk" again. So Paul lost his only source of pleasure and retreated into his barren world of loneliness and desolation.

In the beginning of his stay Paul spoke of leaving the Manor, but no one made an effort to remove him and to find him independent lodgings. He was shunted aside and told to wait, "your time will come." The nursing home would not let him go since his railroad pension together with another small pension brought them a good income. Thus Paul Fenster will never leave his prison and will remain a dependent abused child until his last breath.

Case 3

Mrs. Smith sat in her rocker by the large window in her room with the sunlight streaming in, a magazine in her gnarled hands, her thin, wrinkled, classical face almost grimacing as she read and nodded alternately. Mrs. Smith was surrounded by a few precious possessions which she had been permitted to keep and which were the last remnants of all she had accumulated over her 80 years. There was a very old mahogany rolltop desk which crowded one corner of the double room, a non-playing portable TV set, a porcelain bird on top of the desk and a few plastic plants on the wide window sill; oh yes, and an empty fruit basket, a reminder that she loved fresh fruit and had received some for Christmas from her roommate's family. Except for a severe hearing loss Mrs. Smith was remarkably alert and appeared to know everything that was in the daily news and a great deal about other things as well.

Mrs. Smith had lost her husband when she was in her fifties, then had moved to Florida with a friend who gave her a job as seamstress. She lived there for a number of years until her last remaining sister became ill and needed her services. She rented an apartment in Buffalo and lived with Mrs. Houseman, her invalid sister, until she herself had an emotional breakdown two years ago. Then she was taken to a local hospital and from there transferred to the Manor, the nursing home in which she now lived, and where her sister died a year earlier. Her life's savings of $12,000 had dwindled to nothing within the year, she was told, but she received no accounting of this. Her lawyer and a great niece who had been appointed guardian never came to visit. Toward the end of the first year the nursing home no longer gave her the $28.50 due her from Social Security, claiming that she owed them more than they could ever extract from her. The little remaining joy that she had known, namely, being taken to a restaurant by a distant friend, could no longer be done since Mrs. Smith had no funds to pay for this. Her shoes began to wear out and the few dresses she had in her possession were threadbare and mended too many times. Even her hearing aid batteries were beginning to be used up and the nursing home proprietress ignored her requests for new ones. "You use up more than we can give you, lady," an emissary of the proprietress would snarl. Thus Mrs. Smith attempted to read lips and was shut out from the world of hearing. She was afraid to protest for fear she would be removed from these familiar surroundings to an even worse situation. At least here she knew the aides who hadn't left since she came. She had already bribed some of the help with some of her former possessions, hoping this would assure her a place in the Manor for the remainder of her life.

Although she had been one of eight children there was no one left to whom she could turn. Her great niece who had once shown a trifle of interest did not come to see her since her money had been exhausted. Daily Mrs. Smith waited for some word from the outside world, a glimmer of hope and recognition of friends whom she had met over the years and who might remember her.

Although she walked not too fast she had no debilitating disease and became a prisoner of the nursing home because of lack of interest, relatives or money. The social worker who had spent forty-five minutes a week with her could do nothing except listen, since the establishment refused to keep anyone with an interest in bettering the patients' lot. Mrs. Smith begged the worker to say nothing to anyone about her problems and one day her last ear, the social worker, was discharged "due to lack of funds."

Mrs. Smith will forever watch the spring, winter, summer and autumn from within her room, looking out the window until she becomes so depressed that she will either be removed to a state institution or strapped to a bed in isolation, drugged until her once clear mind will wander into the abyss of total insanity.

Case 4

An attractive white haired handsome woman of 91 sat erectly in a wheelchair. Her resolute countenance showed the determination to live. She must have been stately and tall only a few months earlier. Her speech was clear and coherent as she told of her life. She had come to the nursing home in December of 1971, upon the insistence of her wealthy granddaughter. Mrs. Ferguson's husband had died suddenly in Florida and in her grief she had returned to Buffalo where her closest family members lived. These were a well-to-do couple in their middle years who were childless themselves and who did not want the "responsibility of grandma" in their elegant $60,000 suburban home. Mrs. Ferguson's only child had died when he was only 26 leaving one child, the granddaughter, behind. Mrs. Ferguson had doted on this youngster and helped her in many ways until the young woman was married to a wealthy man.

Orders had been given to the nursing home by the woman's physician that she was to be harnessed into her wheelchair and tied to her bed lest she fall "and break a hip." She had only fallen once because a leaking water faucet at the nursing home had formed a puddle on the floor in which the "patient" slipped. She had received only a few contusions and had walked away without any serious injuries. The nursing home had been told that if they unharnessed Mrs. Ferguson they would be promptly sued. Mrs. Ferguson's muscles were becoming more and more rigid from disuse due to the forced idleness of her limbs. Mrs. Ferguson was experiencing pain and swelling as she was not allowed to stand. She unstrapped herself on one occasion and was duly disciplined by being tightly strapped into her bed, leaving marks where the restraints had cut into her flesh.

The grandson had visited Mrs. Ferguson once and had her sign over the power of attorney to him, and had also appointed his cousin to be the attorney for the patient's estate. All the pleas of Mrs. Ferguson that another attorney be contacted were of no avail. Her family promised to do so, popped a piece of candy in her mouth and went away with no intention of doing anything of the sort. Mrs. Ferguson asked to return to Florida where she could be her own person and be in charge of her own life. All she received were shrugs and complacent, meaningless patronizing. Mrs. Ferguson is a prisoner of her caretakers and will never see the outside of her prison again.

Case 5

Mrs. Flesher, or Claudia as she was known to the staff of the nursing home, has the appearance of an old Madonna. Her blue eyes still sparkle occasionally although often through tears. Her snow-white hair is covered by a thin hair net and her strikingly handsome face is lined with wrinkles. She spends most of the day in her wheelchair when she isn't curled up in bed with her hands under her face.

Mrs. Flesher cannot remember names and she addresses people as "Yoo-hoo." With much effort she is able to recollect certain situations in her life, especially those that were most painful to her. She clings to thoughts about "Mama," a thought which serves "The Rescue Function" for her in her bleak existence. Mrs. Flesher was one of eight children, of whom only one sister remains. Her mother had a very difficult existence since her husband, Mrs. Flesher's father, was a tailor who drank rather heavily. At a fairly young age Claudia married her husband John and they had one son, Richard. After the death of her husband Claudia lived with her son and his second wife. She had raised her granddaughter, Bonnie, since Richard's first wife had died when Bonnie was only three years old. After fourteen months of living with her son, the daughter-in-law decided that she could no longer tolerate Claudia and she went from the hospital to the nursing home. In the beginning of her stay Mrs. Flesher was lucid and hopeful that she would return "home" but as the months went by all hope left Claudia and she began to lose her memory for current events - eventually even past events.

Her body ached from head to toe but the nurses just passed her by since she could not express herself clearly and they did not care. They did not take the trouble to find out why her face was distorted with pain. She looked much like a helpless child searching for relief through her dirt-speckled glasses. Since she was unable to approach the nurses, her bowel impaction went unnoticed and she suffered with a quiet, almost per-sistent, moan of "MMMMMMM!" The aides would occasionally rush by her with "you'll be allright, Claudia!"

When Mrs. Flesher was brought to the nursing home her son Richard confiscated her bank accounts and other assets which Mr. and Mrs. Flesher had painstakingly accumulated over the years. She became very much aware of this situation and hardly wanted to see him when he visited for five minutes once a week. The granddaughter whom she had raised was resentful of the wheelchair which Richard had been half coerced to purchase for her. For weeks she did not visit nor bring the three great-grandsons who meant so much to Claudia. Mrs. Flesher's roommate is a total care case whose TV is ceaselessly turned on from morning to night. Although this is very disturbing to Claudia the nursing home staff has ignored her pleas which are expressed in half spoken sentences.

Mrs. Flesher wants to die. "No you don't" is the reply she receives when she manages to express her desperation in that fashion. Mrs. Flesher will die, a welcome relief from the living death which is now hers.

Case 6

Until she was thirty years old, Mrs. Amelia Hathaway took care of her elderly mother, for her mother was a widow and not too well. One evening she went to a local bar for a beer where she met Frank whom she married a few days later. She soon learned that her husband was an alcoholic. It was extremely difficult living with him. After two years Amelia became pregnant, miscarried and was promptly deserted by her spouse. She then returned to live with her mother, obtained a job as governess and supported her mother and herself on her small earnings. When the mother died ten years later, Mrs. Hathaway became a full time "live-in servant" for two families, one after the other, raising six children, all told.

Over the years Mrs. Hathaway noticed that her walking became difficult and that her hands were beginning to show signs of gnarling. A local doctor diagnosed her condition as one of a severe case of osteo-arthritis, predicting that this would eventually lead to total crippling and immobility. The prediction came true.

In her neighborhood was a nursing home called the Wheel which housed 90 wheelchair bound patients. One day she decided to look it over and to ask the administrator whether she could be considered for residency since she desperately needed care. She agreed to give the institution her worldly possessions in exchange for asylum for the remainder of her life.

She was very interested in the current gossip and made herself important to the staff and administration by carrying stories about the other patients to them. She always praised her keepers and told them interesting stories of her youth, her foster children and her alcoholic husband. She became increasingly more debilitated until she became a total care patient and had to be washed, toileted and fed. The staff loved her. One 16 year old Aide brought her cookies from home and showered her with affection. The young Aide was almost unaware of Amelia's condition until a visitor came in and remarked that Mrs. Hathaway looked like a "vegetable." The Aide made Mrs. Hathaway her pet. She peeled her grapes and tomatoes, etc. To the Aides Mrs. Hathaway was wonderful and nice with a warmth that only she could give. The patient gave such vivid descriptions when she spoke that one could almost taste the Russell Stover candies which seemed so important to the frail elderly lady. Mrs. Hathaway waited from one meal to the other always wondering out loud, yet always knowing, what would be served next. She knew the life history of every patient and how many visitors they had per week. Mrs. Hathaway herself had few visitors; only at Christmas time did she hear from her former wards who would send her greetings and candy. Mrs. Hathaway had a toothless mouth since there was no money to pay for dentures. She would endlessly suck on candy in her reclining position.

She was placed on the welfare rolls since the nursing home felt they could not keep her without financial assistance. Mrs. Hathaway had next to no spending money and depended on the good will of the Aides to supply her with a few sweets which she craved. She had wonderful vision and could spot anything that came into her periphery many feet away. She was very perceptive and would notice the wrong-doing of the staff who were not performing properly. One middle aged Aide would constantly disappear into the bathroom. Mrs. Hathaway was fully aware of this. She also noticed that a retarded Aide dealt with her very roughly and hurt her ailing body.

On occasion Mrs. Hathaway would weep quietly into her pillow because she felt so inadequate and couldn't feed herself. When she was moved to the second floor where the very sick patients were she sobbed loudly for hours knowing that this was the last station before the cemetery. (It was the practice of the Wheel to move dying patients to the second floor.) Mrs. Hathaway loved life however and she clung to it for two more years before she quietly expired in her sleep.

Case 7

Annie O'Neill was an immigrant from Ireland who had come over to
Canada with her three children some 40 years ago. Soon after her arrival
her husband passed away and she had to raise her young family all by herself. She did housework for various people and took her children with her
whenever she could. As the youngsters came of school age she moved to
America where she had a friend - an Irish woman who had come from the old
country about the same time that she had. When her children were grown
she was able to save enough money to have a small place of her own where
she planted beautiful flowers and kept a small vegetable garden. As is
the fate of so many parents her children moved away from Buffalo and she
was left alone. Although she worked hard all of her life, cleaning
peoples' houses and catering to their needs, her financial situation was a
meager one. Her children were having families and were unable to do much
more than visit her occasionally and send her letters from out of town.
Annie was a beautiful woman with snow-white hair and twinkling blue eyes,
and a delightful Irish brogue that would catch anyone's ear.

As she got older she became more and more forgetful and had a difficult time doing her housework. Occasionally she would forget to turn the
gas off after she finished cooking. One day her oldest daughter came to
visit her and decided that her mother should be taken care of in a nursing
home. She consulted with her two siblings who were only too glad to initiate the move to have her institutionalized. The daughter told Annie
wonderful stories of how she would be living in a resort-like place with

no cooking to be done, no one to worry about and that all of her minor and major physical cares would be handled. The daughter also convinced Mrs. O'Neill that her few meager possessions would be written into her own name so that she could hand her money whenever necessary. Mrs. O'Neill wanted to believe all that her child had told her. When the day came for her to leave her small abode she wept, said goodbye to her neighbors and shed a few tears but, after all, she was going to "Shangri-la" and there was no real need to be sad.

The daughter accompanied her to Country Palace - a large air-conditioned nursing home far away from Buffalo, inaccessible to everyone whom she had known. Her daughter bade her farewell and was not seen again. Her boys wrote polite letters reassuring her that she was now safe and happy and that there was no better place for her.

Annie sat day in and day out watching patients wheel up the hall, wondering what would be on the breakfast, lunch and dinner menus. Her outgoing personality and winning smile soon caused others in the Home to befriend her and to seek her out. One elderly gentleman and she began to exchange nursery rhymes and Annie's melodious voice would rin in the dining room, "I hope you live till a dead horrse kicks you." "Hickory dickory dock - the mouse went up the clock," chimed in her gentleman friend. "Herre's a spoon," twittered Annie. A cow jumped "over" the moon, answered her friend. These two people soon gathered a small audience around them every morning, and inadvertently they would entertain the other inmates of Country Palace.

Annie would eat ravenously and wait from one meal to another. She could never get enough food. She often reminisced about the Irish famine and with that she would smack her lips and take a couple more slices of toast off another patient's plate.

As time went on Annie became less and less lucid, speaking more and more in rhymes. If asked what she planned to do with her future she would speak in nonsense syllables. Eventually she would say, "My children love me. They come to see me every day." She turned the love which she craved into a phantasy which seemed very real to her. Annie will be lost in her own little world forever.

Case 8

Mr. Anton Santolido was a 78 year old gentleman who had come to Haven Manor a year after his wife's death which occurred two years ago. He had raised two successful sons by working in his small shoe repair shop. A minor stroke necessitated hospitalization and his eventual transfer to the Haven. Both of his sons' wives were employed and there was no one to take care of him in his own apartment.

Mr. Santolido was very lonely at the Haven and he very much missed the affection that his wife had lavished on him for more than 50 years. His English was not too polished or clear which did not help Anton with the other residents. He was not a literate man, thus he was left to his own devices much of the time. He attempted to approach others and to hold conversations with them but since no one in the Manor spoke Italian they turned their backs on him and ignored him.

One day he forced a kiss upon the cheek of a female patient who had the room across the hall from him. After that he became known as "the dirty old man" and was restrained in his bed whenever he went to his room. "The next thing you know he'll molest someone", the aides quipped. After this episode Mr. Santolido regressed more and more. Since he was so often confined and had nothing to look toward, no highlights, only the drab imprisonment of the Manor with its restraints, he mumbled to himself in unintelligible sounds. One day when no one was very near and when they had forgotten to "strap him in", he crawled into bed with a babbling female patient. The staff eventually discovered him there as he called this woman by his wife's name and tried to make love to her.

The treatment of Mr. Santolido after that became progressively worse. He was only allowed to go to the dining room to have his three meals a day and the remainder of the time he was strapped into a chair in the television lounge or in his room. There was talk about "shipping him out" but there was no institution that would readily accept him. The State Hospital in the area was approached and a team of "experts" came to visit Mr. Santolido. They determined that he did not need hospitalization and thus other arrangements would need to be made for him.

Mr. Santolido was not a violent man; on the contrary, he was a loving human being who had been cut off from all avenues of gaining and giving affection. He had really reacted in a quite normal fashion for a person who is not confined to an institution. The longer he was confined the greater his frustration became.

When his sons were notified of the situation they gave permission to the Manor to do whatever needed to be done since they did not feel that they could cope with this man of whom they had now become ashamed. They made it clear that they wanted to be disassociated from him.

Anton Santolido is still living at the Haven. What his future will be one can only guess. He will no doubt remain there until he deteriorates completely.

Case 9

Orpha, a 76 year old woman, meandered down the green carpeted nursing home corridor clutching a primitively constructed yarn doll. Occasionally she would spit on the floor and mumble something indistinquishable. Then again she would scream at the doll, clutching it closer to her bosom, "You've been a bad baby, a very bad baby, you've been caught and I'll not let you go." The doll was the only thing that Orpha could have as hers - the only thing that she could control. Her destiny was in the hands of the nursing home overseers. The spitting was the only way that she could show her anger.

Whenever a staff person would leave the nursing home she would question him in a childlike manner, her innocent grey eyes looking him straight in the face: "Where are you going? Why are you going? Why can't I go?" There usually was no reply and the large wooden doors would quickly close behind the employee.

"Who am I?" This she would quickly answer with "me, me, me, me." No history accompanied Orpha except that she had no living relatives, a severe case of diabetes and hardening of the arteries.

Occasionally she would place her worn out doll on the piano and play some nostalgic melodies of years gone by - the last signs, the last remnants of a cultured lady who probably once had loving parents who had cared for their little girl. Often she would jump up from the piano bench, take packets of sugar from the dining room tables, tear open a corner and pour their contents into her mouth - "and none for your baby" she would say to her doll throwing the empty papers around her toy child.

Every day the same ritual takes place until one day Orpha will take her final steps down the long corridor of the Manor.

Case 10

Paula Panka had married at an early age and had three daughters in relatively brief succession. Her husband was a factory laborer who became ill after ten years of marriage and was hospitalized in a nearby State Hospital where he is still an inmate. Mrs. Panka had a difficult time on her meager welfare check, sewed all of her girls' own clothes, kept their small apartment in immaculate order, cooked nourishing, inexpensive meals and had almost none of the ordinary pleasures of life that most people enjoy. She liked watching her daughters grow but hated having to deny them the things that other children had so readily available to them.

Before her marriage she worked as a salesclerk for a local department store and turned over most of her funds to her parents who were extremely poor too. Her whole life was one of financial deprivation and emotional barrenness.

All three of her children had unsuccessful marriages; two married alcoholics and one an unemployed laborer whom she divorced two years after the marriage. The youngest used to confiscate Paula's Social Security check when her mother was not at home. Paula never reported this since she had very strong convictions about parents having loyalty to children "come what may."

At age 60 Paula suffered a stroke and was taken by ambulance to a local hospital. She remained there several weeks and participated in physical therapy; however her whole left side remained paralyzed and limp. The hospital social service department contacted Paula's children and one of them agreed to take her home. This relationship lasted less than a year. Marlene felt that her mother's presence caused her to lose her unborn child during the eighth month of pregnancy since she had to help her in and out of bed. Marlene's alcoholic husband ushered Mrs. Panka out of the house and let her know that she was unwanted and unloved. Mrs. Panka knew that she could not take care of herself. She telephoned the hospital which had released her and was told that they could contact various nursing homes for her until they would find an opening.

Mrs. Panka ended up at Country Manor, a beautifully air-conditioned one-floor unit. She was given a single room but was soon moved to one which had another occupant. Mrs. Panka's children did not visit her for the first three months. They did write a little note stating that the place was too far for them to reach and that their cars were too old to take the risk of traveling an hour away from the city.

Paula learned to smile pleasantly and to say that everything is just perfect. She yearned to see her children and grandchildren but they never came. She did not even receive her Social Security checks of which $24.50 belonged to her for spending money and the remainder to the institution. She verbalized that she knew there must be some mistake and that her children couldn't possibly be withholding her funds. In the meantime she had no allowance to have her hair done, to buy the few cigarettes she craved nor so much as a candy bar or gum. The social worker noticed the patient's dilemma and contacted the youngest daughter, insisting that her Social Security checks be mailed to her at once. With this threat hanging over the girl's head the checks began to come in and Mrs. Panka could buy the few items which she so much wanted and enjoyed.

Mrs. Panka needed dentures but when the administrator was approached the staff was informed that if Mrs. Panka didn't take care of her teeth in her youth she needn't think that she would get handouts now. Without the administrator's permission the county could not be contacted for teeth for this patient. For months Mrs. Panka lived on cereals, liquids and toast soaked in coffee or tea. Finally a nurse who was very fond of this patient saved and collected money to enable Paula to be fitted for dentures.

Occasionally Paula would request to be placed into a nursing home nearer her children. When the administrator heard of this she became very angry and threatened to fire the social worker who had agreed to find such a place for Paula because Paula had gone to the administrator to tell her of her plans. After this Paula became totally submissive and subservient and claimed that she loved Country Manor and did not want to be anywhere else on earth. Paula is getting her wish. If Paula remains in reasonably good health and causes no problems, makes no waves and praises the administrator and minor administrative officials, she can stay in the Manor and smile until she becomes ill. Then she will be evicted, to smile elsewhere, submissive, silent and condemned to suffer for the crime of being old.

Case 11

Miss Post looked like a tall unfortunate child, with a very sad face, gaunt features and a very thin body, as she slowly wended her way down the long waxed hall of the nursing floor corridors leaning heavily on her walker. Her expression was one of hopelessness. She was a 70 year old woman who had worked as a bookkeeper for the railroad all of her life and who had lived with her aging parents in their small middle class home. When the last of her parents, her father, died, she became depressed and was treated with shock therapy at a hospital. At the request of a distant cousin she was transferred from there to the nursing home. She was constantly preoccupied with paying her bills which were mounting to astronomical proportions; she had realistic fears of losing her house and wanted an answer and an exact accounting of her possessions. She asked many questions of the nursing home manager, but was brushed off and told not to worry. Nevertheless, she had to send checks every month and her bank balance diminished very rapidly. She was asked to sign for the selling of her home. She protested feebly that she did not want to do this as she was expecting to return to her home, but to no avail. Three people surrounded her: the manager, the head nurse and her distant cousin, and ordered her to sign "the papers." With a shaky, scrawly handwriting she signed away her last earthly possessions. After this episode panic struck. She asked again what was going to happen to her and she was told, "you'll be allright." No valid answer was forthcoming. She couldn't eat, had no funds to buy anything and became weaker and weaker. She began looking at her hands and mumbling to herself. Occasionally she would scream out "help me, help me!", because help was what she truly needed. She became more and more transparent and finally was too weak to get out of bed. She cared nothing about her appearance and although she had wept a great deal in the beginning she became apathetic. Only when the aides came to toilet her did she occasionally cry in a pain-like wail and at other times she would scratch at her caretakers. The staff finally dubbed her as "paranoid" and isolated her in a room all by herself, with the door almost closed all day. She could not reach the bell when she needed help so her weak cries were unheeded. Her very sensible requests turned into garbled unrealities as she lay in bed day after day in a semi-stuporous state without visitors and without love. It will not be long before Miss Post's frail body will cease to be and will join her mind in the hereafter, if one there be.

Case 12

Mrs. Deerberg was a large pleasant looking woman with roughhewn features. She lived alone in her colonial home except for the summer when her 92 year old aunt would come from Florida to be with her. Barbara's husband had died two years earlier after a lingering illness. She and her husband were a team - extremely close. They had married late in life - when Mrs. Deerberg was in her forties. Her husband took on the responsibility of her ailing brother who also shared their home until his death some ten years ago. Mr. and Mrs. Deerberg enjoyed traveling, playing cards and visiting with neighbors.

One morning Mrs. Deerberg attempted to get up but had a numbing sensation in her head along with an extremely severe headache. She could not make her legs do what she wanted. She was able to reach the telephone to call her niece - a woman who was only 13 years younger than Barbara. A physician was called and Mrs. Deerberg was taken to the hospital with the diagnosis of cerebro-vascular accident. She had suffered a stroke. For three months she lay helplessly in the hospital. With physical therapy and a great deal of medication she was able to walk and regain the use of her limbs. There were no visible signs of debility. She did now tire very quickly however and her doctor ordered her to use a walker forever. The fear of falling was real and she appeared to need the support of an appliance to give her the courage to walk. After several more months in the hospital and with no one at home to take care of her, Mrs. Deerberg was transferred to the nursing home. Her niece explained to the doctor that she already was taking care of the patient's sister and could not take care of another person. The doctor talked to the patient and convinced her that the only place where she would be physically safe would be the Haven. Reluctantly Mrs. Deerberg allowed herself to be convinced.

As she was moved into the Haven on a stretcher she could see high ceilings, hear voices of staff laughing and joking; antiseptic smells mingled with the flavor of cooking reached her nostrils. "That's the patient from the Memorial," a voice was heard calling. The voice directed the aides to push her into a room on the first floor. She later learned that the first floor was for "private pay" patients only. Mrs. Deerberg soon learned that acquiescing and smiling were very important; that they were the way to be liked by the staff. The dignified lady who once was now became the "good girl" of 75. To request too much or to ring the buzzer for the help was an unpardonable sin and one could get moved to a four-bed room for that. She learned to precede minor requests with "if it isn't too much trouble" and to praise the nursing home, its administrator and staff in sweeping grandeur. Mrs. Sickel, the administrator, was spoken of as a "darling," the head nurse became a "dear," the aides were "sweethearts" and the cooks did their very best.

On occasion the patient became panic stricken and needed reassurance that she would not be sent with the more senile patients to the third floor or be thrown out altogether. These reassurances were mostly asked for when other patients were moved for no apparent reason. Mrs.

Deerberg sensed that when people's money ran out they were asked to be removed to a public institution or taken to a dormitory in Haven Manor. Mrs. Deerberg also learned to bribe the staff with cookies and candy bought and brought to her by her niece. At Christmas time she had red and white bells crocheted for all the important staff members - namely all of those who had a great deal of contact with her.

Mrs. Deerberg's niece visited her twice a week but made it progressively clear that she would have to remain in the nursing home until the end of her days. The doctor was also informed by the niece that her aunt was not to be permitted to be taken out of the institution on visits - not even for a day.

There were occasions when Barbara would stay in her room and weep most of the day but afterwards would apologize for expressing feelings and beg the significant staff not to reveal her upset to the administrator nor to her niece lest she lose favor in their eyes and become even more disadvantaged.

Mrs. Deerberg's present and future goal was to be able to keep her room in Haven Manor at any and all costs to herself.

Case 13

Miss Standish is afflicted with "Parkinson's syndrome." She is a very quiet former teacher who socializes very little. She appears to be lost in her own thoughts and forgotten dreams of yesteryear. She was a spinster all of her life and liked teaching her class of first graders.

Shortly after her retirement Miss Standish became ill and was transferred from the hospital into the nursing home. When she first came she was able to walk without assistance but as time wore on she became more unsteady and needed a walker for balance.

Being an educated, cultured woman, Miss Standish had had many experiences on trips to Europe and other events. The other residents ignored her fascinating adventures which she would occasionally share. Thus she became progressively more silent and introspective. She would spend hours merely staring in front of herself through eyes partially covered with cataracts. One day she was told that within a week her eyes would be operated on and she would be able to see. The operation took place but Miss Standish was even less able to see. Only now she had pain in her operated eye and it was perpetually red. Her anxiety over this could be seen in her terrified stare as staff and others passed her. She knew that no one cared, "so there's no point in complaining." She was treated with more patronizing than one would the students whom she taught a few years before.

This once proud woman was thus reduced into a young child with no outlet for her insecurity, ability and need for emotional as well as physical support. Her feeble efforts to find out her condition went unheeded - like a weak unheard voice in a strong wind.

All of this patient's money has now been exhausted and she is tolerated on "Medicaide." She must share her room with three others, one bed fairly close to the next with no autonomy for the comfort of each patient and with no privacy to engage in the natural bodily functions.

Miss Standish suppresses whatever she can at the expense of great physical and emotional pain to herself. She can be seen deteriorating steadily and will one day be carried out in a pine box to her eternal reward.

Case 14

The room suddenly spun wildly around Ileen Weidner. She could not think; even her name was blurred from her mind. A sharp horrible pain permeated Mrs. Weidner's total existence until she fell unconscious to the floor. It was there that she was discovered by a young neighbor and friend who was in the habit of taking her grocery shopping every Friday.

Mrs. Weidner had experienced several life times during her 62 years. When she was 21 years old she came to the U.S. from Marisch-Ostrow (Czechoslovakia) to marry a 33 year old man whom she had known in Europe. She had come from a wealthy home where a bell would bring a servant to do her bidding. In America life was different for her and she had to live in a small flat which she shared with her brother and sister-in-law. She neither knew how to cook or clean and her only talent was music - she possessed a beautiful voice. This was of little help to her since her singing was not a marketable skill.

After her first child was born, she and her husband moved into their own apartment. Five years later a second son was born and the family's financial straits appeared even more acute. She had an unhappy life. Her husband's interests were quite different from hers, partially because of a large age difference and also because of his disinterest in anything musical. He worked hard as a technical chemist, was out of work some of the time and eventually turned to selling novelties from store to store.

When Ileen was 40, her older and favorite son was killed in the second World War and with him went her dreams. She became morose and grudgingly raised her second boy to maturity. Hans moved out of town for college purposes as soon as he was of age. When Ileen was 60 her husband died leaving her all alone. She had never formed close relationship ties so that she could not really turn to anyone in her grief. She was terribly lonely and afraid. Every night was spent in terror that someone would break in and rob her of her few earthly possessions or maim or kill her.

When her neighbor discovered her on the floor she telephoned her son, a professor who lived a long distance away from Buffalo. He promised to fly home two days later but in the meanwhile her only brother was telephoned and he appeared several hours later, as did her physician. Her condition was diagnosed as a cardio-vascular accident. She was transported on a stretcher to the hospital against her will. With a slurred voice she begged to stay in her own home, to no avail. She heard the siren of the ambulance as it sped down her street, to Main Street toward the dreaded hospital. She was strapped onto the stretcher grossly uncomfortable and unable to move. She believed herself to be dying and cried out for her son who was nowhere in sight. The bright lights of the hospital glared ominously down as Ileen looked up from her stretcher. She was transferred to a cot and there lay for many hours until an intern shone a flashlight into her face and asked her some simple questions which she hardly understood. Terror filled her heart until she fell into a restless sleep filled with nightmares.

When her son arrived from the West Coast she clung to him, looked at him beseechingly and begged to be taken with him. He promised to take her back with him but week followed week and his promise was not kept. He returned to work and a month later he came only to admit his mother to a local nursing home. This was a horrible blow to Mrs. Weidner. She could not accept her son's indifference. Her speech became more and more garbled, yet she was aware of her confusion and frequently wept over her inability to make herself understood. Her incoherence gave the staff the opportunity to ignore her and on several occasions she soiled her clothing because they overlooked her pleas to be walked to the toilet. This was very humiliating to a lady who had always been extremely clean. When she asked for orange juice she was given grape or prune - no one paid attention to her wants. She was now "personna non grata" - an individual whose existence or lack of existence seemed to matter to no one. She was a $700 monthly check to the nursing home proprietor.

Mrs. Weidner still lived in the faint hope that her son would some day come to her rescue. One day he did come to remove her bodily to a permanent, much cheaper nursing home, "an old age home." There she aged very rapidly; became blind within a matter of days, "had to be" strapped into a wheelchair and untied herself continuously, muttering and screaming intermittently. The proprietors of this home would not keep her and transferred her to the State Hospital where she died on a ward of 20 beds within a month.

"Ruth Bales died yesterday morning," the social work aide whispered to the consultant.

Mrs. Bales was a refined, genteel lady who always answered the question regarding her well being, "Can't complain." She would remark on the weather and how "the good Lord" watches over everyone. Mrs. Bales was placed in Recovery Haven by her daughter who was very critical of her and who felt hampered by this 77 year old woman's existence. She furthermore felt that she could not have the kind of social life she wanted as the wife of a dentist when her mother's mere presence constantly reminded her of her financially meager past. Mama could not understand the rejection, especially since she had her very own room and bath on the third floor of the daughter's spacious mansion-like home. The son-in-law and daughter stopped off at Recovery Haven and left her there saying that she needed a little rest. Mrs. Bales was too stunned to say too much. Tears rolled down her cheeks and her saucer-like eyes which appeared even bigger through her very thick lenses were red and swollen by the end of that endless day.

Although Ruth had had a wonderful memory she almost instantly forgot how she had gotten to the Haven but did remember her childhood and growing up years with surprising vividness. Mrs. Bales was raised by two "good Christian parents" in a family of seven children. Her father had taken them for long walks on Sundays and in the afternoon, had played games with them; he suddenly disappeared and one child or the other always gleefully found him, much to the others' "surprise" and delight. He would tell them amusing stories and entertain his children for hours. In the meantime Ruth's mother had the opportunity to nap since "she was a small bitty woman and so very good." The parents got along very well together. There was not much money to go around but everyone ate well and appeared fairly contented. The mother was an excellent cook and the father brought home his paycheck religiously for the mother to manage.

Ruth married a working man when she was in her early twenties and did the housewifely chores as well as raising three children: two sons and a daughter. She followed pretty much in her mother's footsteps. She sewed her children's clothes, cooked, baked, went to church with her family until they reached adulthood. Her spouse died when she was 64 and between her meager savings and her Social Security check she was able to get along. Her two sons moved out of town to take jobs and her daughter urged her to sell her home and move into a cramped apartment. The mother finally allowed herself to be convinced.

Apartment living did not agree with Ruth and she missed her small yard and flower beds. Daughter Martha then suggested that Ruth move in with her, thus they could "share" expenses and it would be cheaper for them both. Soon the daughter managed to get power of attorney. A few years thereafter Mother entered Recovery Haven.

Although the daughter visited the Haven weekly, the mother could not remember the visits for more than a day after Martha and her husband had been there. The two out of town sons wrote to Ruth occasionally.

Life in the Haven was very monotonous for Ruth. She would get up, dress and use her cane to get to the dining room an hour before breakfast was served. She would sit patiently and fold and refold the napkins on her table, the table she shared with two very senile women. The staff paid very little attention to Ruth since she demanded nothing and made a smiling grimace every time one of them passed by. "Ruthy, Ruthy, yessee, yessee" one young aide used to say laughingly. The others would claim among themselves that Ruth was very happy in the nursing home.

The real Ruth no one understood. She ruminated all day about what she might have done to deserve her fate and then would reminisce with the social work consultant about her childhood, especially adulating her father who she wished was alive to rescue her now from her dilemma.

One day Ruth fell out of bed attempting to reach her cane. She fractured her hip and was moved to the local hospital, but soon returned to Recovery Haven where she stopped eating and died a week thereafter. When Martha was notified of her mother's death she appeared within the hour demanding the $15 which her mother had "stashed away for a rainy day." It would never rain on Ruth again.

Case 16

Ellen was married at a very early age to Jason Ullman. She was 16 and he was 23. Mr. Ullman never earned much money since he was a grade school drop-out who became a dish washer and restaurant helper. The couple had one son and the three lived on Mr. Ullman's meager income in a small upstairs apartment. Mrs. Ullman was a good cook and homemaker and enjoyed sewing curtains and other things to make her home look presentable and comfortable. When their son reached the age of 18 he joined the Armed Forces and did not come home except for furloughs. Although the Ullmans were a devoted couple, the shortage of money in the home sometimes made one of the others cross and life was rather thorny at times.

At age 50 Mrs. Ullman suffered a stroke. Her husband found her on the floor when he came home from work. Not having a doctor or a car, he called to his downstairs neighbor and together they transported Ellen to the nearest hospital. The stay in the county hospital was a long and trying one. Mrs. Ullman was placed on the ward with many other "welfare" patients. Her condition appeared to be getting progressively worse. After three months her vision was so poor that she had to wear dark glasses in order to see at all. She needed a wheelchair for ambulation and at times her speech was garbled. Her speech problem eventually cleared up but she knew she would never walk again, or eat totally unassisted.

The hospital's social service worker called on the husband and asked him to have his wife transferred to a nursing home since they needed the bed and could no longer keep Ellen. With the worker's help a place was found for Mrs. Ullman in the country - an hour's drive from the big city. Mr. Ullman in his desperation accepted the spot although he knw that he would probably rarely see his wife again since he had no means of transportation. Soon after Mrs. Ullman's transfer to the nursing home, Mr. Ullman suffered a mild heart attack and was told he could never work again.

In the nursing home Mrs. Ullman was the picture of unhappiness. She yearned to see and talk to her Jason and dreamed of a time when her son would be discharged from the service and take care of herself and her spouse. She begged the nursing home personnel to have her transferred to Buffalo so that she could see her husband but they ignored her and treated her with disdain.

The situation of Ellen Ullman came to the attention of the nursing home social worker. Painstakingly Ellen told her of her plight. She told of the many lonely hours that she was spending, how she couldn't sleep at night and how much she wanted to see her husband before her vision would be completely gone. She understood that she had no one to live with but said that she would be satisfied just living in another nursing home in Buffalo near her husband. The social worker telephoned many nursing homes in Buffalo until she found one with a vacancy which was willing to take a welfare patient on "Medicaide." When this action came to the attention of the nursing home administrator she first called in Mrs. Ullman, told her she was an ungrateful cripple who had no rights since she could pay for nothing. She next ushered the social worker into her office with the threat to fire her if this or any other patient were moved from the premises. After this, people were very abrupt with Ellen. She received less and less care as the aides were fearful of being seen doing too much for this patient.

One evening the social worker telephoned Mr. Ullman and advised
him to begin procedures to move his wife into a Buffalo nursing home.
When Mrs. Ullman was moved after many months and through the efforts
of her spouse, the social worker's job was reduced to a part-time position.

PART III

Some Critical Issues in the Treatment
of Nursing Home Patients

1. Abandonment:

Whether we consult the literature concerning nursing home patients, such as Claire Townsend's excellent volume, <u>The Last Segregation</u>, or talk to patients or employees, there is universal agreement that the most painful, the most severe and the most debilitating problem of nursing home patients is abandonment. In fact, we believe that almost all of the other problems which the aged nursing home patient faces, and which range from health care to nutrition and recreation, are intensified, aggravated and sometimes caused by rejection, loneliness and abandonment. Similar problems also face the younger patient, but since rehabilitation and eventual release gives younger patients a future and an evident stake in their society, this problem is not nearly as severe as with the old.

Abandonment has many facets and many variations. Not only those who are abandoned by their families, but also those who had no families, feel the severity of this "last segregation." Familiar streets, familiar houses, cursory acquaintances, the local grocer, the "cop" on the beat, all become an integral part of each of us. As we grow older, these common landmarks spell

out our existence and define our being. Like our name, they

tell us who we are, what role we are to play, what our limits

and our opportunities may be and how we fit into the larger

social group. Therefore, any separation becomes a fearsome

experience for those whose age guarantees that they have no

future and that they face at any moment not only the "last seg-

regation" but death, the "last separation."

As our physical condition deteriorates with age our depen-

dency needs increase. Tasks which were once performed unthink-

ingly become major problems so that our "life space" becomes

restricted to those activities which we can accomplish within

the limits of our remaining powers or which we can have done for

us by paying for them.

The phrase "paying" can of course refer to financial remun-

eration. However, there is another form of payment which exists

in ordinary relationships. This is the "social price." By the

"social price" we mean the favors of a non-material sort which

people do for one another; for instance, helping one another to

gain introductions to other people, locating jobs, helping us

gain admittance to country clubs or colleges, or introducing a

newcomer to the social life of his community. All this, it would

appear, the poor old ager can no longer do. Thus, younger people

do not anticipate that the aged can ever repay them for favors done. Therefore they tend to ignore the old and separate themselves from them, particularly since such separation appears imminent already. The consequence is the development of both ageism and gerontophobia. "Ageism" is defined as the sum of "negative attitudes and practices which discriminate against the aged."[1] While this concept has a limited validity, we support the view of Bunzel who more succinctly speaks of "gerontophobia" which he defines as: "the unreasonable fear or irrational hatred of older people by society and by themselves." This makes "Gerontophobia" a socio-psychological concept as it is rooted in the "life space" of the aged. Thus, Bunzel speaks of "Medical Gerontophobia" which affects doctors, nurses, orderlies, nursing home operators, hospital administrators and others. Then there is "Legal Gerontophobia" which affects legislators, administrators, agency heads and legal personnel such as the police, lawyers, judges, courts and clerks. Finally, Bunzel lists "Social Gerontophobia" which affects anyone and results in every kind of discrimination, insult, avoidance and antagonism to the old.[2]

Evidence that this kind of avoidance reaction is related to status in a social group is mainly derived from accounts of the treatment of older members of society among ancestor worshippers.[3] This pattern was once common among the Japanese and others, but as the extended family declines in industrial societies, the

old no longer have this security.[4] Thus, abandonment is an unan-
ticipated consequence of industrial life which includes high
mobility, small families, economic independence and a need to do
almost everything for oneself. The old cannot do for themselves,
therefore they are abandoned by those whose daily tasks occupy
almost all their own time, their own effort and their own strength.

2. Architecture:

Since most nursing homes are operated as businesses by private
profit enterpreneurs, it is not surprising that a number of such
homes in many cities have been condemned as fire traps, and worse.
These extreme abuses are of course easily visible, and while they
are not uncommon they are most likely to be controlled because they
are glaringly evident.

There are, however, architectural problems related to nursing
homes which are not so visible and which generally escape the observation of those who are not themselves nursing home patients.

Thus, the glare created by glass doors in the lobby of a modern
building often makes it difficult for some of the patients to go
into the lobby because their eyes cannot tolerate the reflection
of sunlight from the doors. Yet this very feature seems an asset
to those younger visitors whose eyes are not so affected.

Carpeting creates another problem. It may look beautiful and
create a sense of warmth and refinement. However, carpets are hard

to keep clean when a part of the nursing home population can be counted on to be incontinent and vomiting is not uncommon.

Safety features of all kinds are needed in nursing homes but are not needed by those who visit them. Hand rails in the halls, in bathing facilities and in bedrooms may not occur to those who do not need them.

3. Admissions:

Perhaps the most critical issue in the life of any American is the decision to enter any institution.

We have already seen that Americans believe passionately in independence and the right to self-determination. We have also seen that those who do not enjoy these rights, for any reason, feel a loss of status within their reference groups, based on internalized values as generally taught in our culture.

Therefore, entrance into a nursing home is particularly traumatic for the aged, since many rightly believe that they will never be independent again and that they will be "carried out in a pine box." Such beliefs are obviously not without foundation. It is therefore of the greatest importance that the decision to enter a nursing home be made by the patient himself, that the decision be made with full knowledge of the facts surrounding a patient's situation, and, most important, that the patient know the nature of the institution he is about to enter. It is our view that generally, that is, in most instances, patients about to be admitted to nursing homes have no such knowledge and that they are almost always inadequately prepared for this momentous step in their lives.

Ordinarily, patients become candidates for entrance to a "Nursing Home" without knowing this. The decision that some-one should enter such a home is generally made by physicians, nurses, hospital administrators and, of course, relatives. The most common situation is one in which an old woman or old man has been in a hospital for an acute illness and the physician has decided to discharge the patient. The patient then believes that he should go home and fully expects to do so. However, it is at this point that his relatives, often his children, decide not to readmit him to his home and to send him to an institu-tion. When a patient has no relatives, or was not living with anyone else before admission to the hospital, the decision to institutionalize is generally made by the attending physicians, nurses and the social service department of the hospital. Most important, however, is the anxiety of hospital administrations to rid themselves of patients whose finances are insufficient to pay the huge charges generally collected for hospital care.

Thus, any patient whose insurance benefits have run out will find that hospital administrators will want him removed at once lest the profits earned by most hospitals on each available bed be reduced. At that point tremendous pressure is exerted upon the sick and old to enter any nursing home just to get out of that hospital bed.

Such "pressure" usually comes as a shock to the patient. This is true first because hospital administrators seldom tell a patient that he can leave when the physician has reached that decision. The information is usually saved until the patient's money has run out. Since this can constitute a time lapse of several weeks, valuable time is lost in which a patient could be given an opportunity to prepare himself for discharge from the hospital and during which he could either make his own arrangements or make arrangements through the efforts of the hospital social service departments. We find, however, that hospital social workers seldom inform patients of their impending discharge and then pressure the poor to sign an admission agreement with a nursing home on the very day, and at the very hour, when they first learned that they are to leave the hospital. In other words, the decision to take the patient to a nursing home is made by others, the patient is given no right to determine his own fate and is largely forced against his will to enter a home which may well appear to him to be a prison from which there is no return. The patient is right all too often.

Since some public institutions have no admissions agreements, patients who are to enter such public homes are asked to

sign a "Medicaid" application which serves the same purpose
since this compensates the public institution as does the
Federal "Supplemental Security Income" for those not covered
by Social Security.

We believe that every institution should have a detailed
admissions agreement; that this agreement should conform to
Federal, State and local laws pertaining to the treatment of
nursing home patients; that a copy of such an agreement should
be given the patient before he enters any institution and that
another copy should be filed with the State Attorney General.
We believe that stringent inspection of all nursing homes, both
public and private, should be made by officers of the Attorney
General in each State with a view to ascertaining that the terms
of these admissions agreements are being scrupulously observed.

An excellent example of this need is the disposition of
the $28.50 allowance which each Social Security Pension recip-
ient must be permitted to retain from pension checks sent
directly to nursing home administrators. A strict accounting of
such funds should be required of all nursing home operators at
least twice a year. In addition, the words "personal allowance"
should be defined in the admissions agreement. Patients should
not only have free access to these funds at will, but the nursing home should be required to include in the agreement a statement concerning expenses for which the patient will not be asked

to pay himself. Thus, a home should have no right to ask a patient to pay for a wheelchair out of his personal allowance which after the patient "leaves" becomes the property of the nursing home.

Rehabilitation begins at admission. This is the minimum professional requirement almost always ignored in practice. The major reason for failure to make good plans is of course poverty. Where resources are lacking, pensions are small and public assistance meager, planning becomes limited to a very few obvious choices. Generally this means that public homes must be used by the poor. As we have already seen, such public homes are generally viewed with fear and are considered ante-chambers to death. Many are called "The Poorhouse" and are dreaded as dumping grounds for the unwanted.

While all this can be the case, we find that public insti-tutions are generally better equipped, better staffed and much more diversified than all but the most expensive private nursing homes. The reasons are of course self evident. Equipment such as whirlpool baths, dental laboratories, and tilt tables cost too much for private operators and are often worthwhile only if the population of the nursing home is large enough to make the investment in trained staff and expensive machines worthwhile. At the same time it must be noted here that large institutions present some serious handicaps, particularly high staff turnover, impersonal treatment and mass cooking and feeding.

4. Food:

In every institution there is a great deal of complaint concerning the nature of the food, its preparation and taste. These complaints have been heard for years in colleges, hospitals, armies, prisons and of course nursing homes. Several reasons for such complaints can be recognized. First, it is frequently true that food is poor and monotonous because the food budget is low. In some institutions, food budgets are higher than is apparent, but administrators save money for themselves or their bosses by spending less on food than they should. In nursing homes, however, additional problems enter into the food complaints. It is evident that no nursing home can deal with a homogeneous population, a fact which faces all institutions. Thus, it would be a miracle if several hundred people, all eating the same food, would find it to their taste. Most everyone is accustomed to something other than that which he must now eat. Everyone remembers home cooking as he knew it and, obviously, institutional cooking approximates only the tastes of a very few. The patient's ethnic food tastes cannot be taken into consideration and that, coupled with his diet, rarely makes the fare palatable. In nursing homes the physical condition of so many patients enters heavily upon the problem. Thus, diets of every kind should be observed but are not. Many old nursing home patients cannot eat various foods because their teeth are faulty, because they suffer from diabetes or other restrictive illnesses or because they cannot tolerate their table mates' eating habits. In addition, some patients cannot reach out and take food from a common supply on their table because of arthritic and other paralytic conditions. Thus they go hungry while more agile table mates eat all there is. This is often too little in any event. We therefore approve the practice of some nursing homes of supplying individual trays of food to each patient. Even when this is done, patients are often ignored when liquids are served by staff aides.

It is therefore recommended that patients seat themselves wherever they please instead of having to sit in assigned seats. Assignment is in any event degrading and insulting to the dignity of adults. It becomes particularly poor policy when it makes eating more difficult. The argument that random selection of seats increases management problems is spurious since nursing employees are appointed for the convenience of the patients, not the other way around. We recognize however that some patients are so attractive that this kind of voluntarism can result in some patients being the only table mates chosen and the subsequent exclusion of others. Food is a very important issue in the lives of nursing home patients. This is true in part because old age forces all of us to be more selective and circumspect with reference to our food habits, but also because food and meals generally become a larger event in the lives of those who have little else to do than to eat because nursing home routines seldom allow patients many other outlets.

In part the monotony of nursing home life is the product of institutionalization itself. In part, however, it is the product of retirement from employment. Few Americans recognize that "retirement begins in childhood" and therefore few are able to deal with it when it suddenly comes upon them at age 65. Those whose life content has been their work find it almost impossible to divorce themselves from such work. They see each day as a monotonous repetition of yesterday and tomorrow as a repetition of today. They blame the nursing home, the food, the administrators, the staff and their whole world. Yet, their own lack of interests, failure to substitute various activities for remunerative work, inability to develop interests in their old age which they did not have in their youth, all contribute to the monotony and the dullness of nursing home existence. In such an environment, food becomes the prime focus in life and therefore the object of every frustration, the butt of every complaint and the center of every difficulty.

It is our view that while the diet problem is often ignored by the food management in nursing homes and while some food complaints are real enough, the chief means of improving the condition of the patients is to focus on daily activities which will decrease interest in food and reduce that interest to a more realistic perspective.

5. The Healer:

The physician rarely visits his patients in the nursing home. He is a figment in the imagination of the patient and a name in the verbiage of the nursing and auxiliary staff. If he has less than three patients in any one nursing home it is hardly worth his while to visit them. The time that he must invest to travel to and from the Home is more remuneratively spent in his office. The doctor prescribes medications on the telephone and often delays return calls indefinitely. If the nursing staff does not notify him of the death of a patient he does not become aware of this. Therefore it often happens that a patient's family is billed for visits from a physician which were never made because the patient was already dead on the date given on the bill for the alleged visit.

When the doctor does visit his patient he generally spends from one to five minutes with him, asks him how he feels and if everyone is good to him. He may say a few comforting words, or tell the patient that his illness will take time. Time indeed, because in time the patient will be dead. One very "fine" physician told his cancer patient that she was going to die very shortly and proceeded to give the details of her final hours, namely, that she might choke. This was so disturbing to the patient that she died soon thereafter of a heart attack.

Thorough examinations are rarely done since the physician takes the attitude that the patient is in the nursing home to die anyway and that therefore there is no point in wasting his valuable time with an aged, very ill, impoverished patient. If the family insists and visits a great deal, and the patient in question is "a private pay" patient, this picture changes and the doctor will make more of an effort to please. The patients imbue the doctor with godlike qualities and quote him incessantly from memory or wishful thinking. They look to him for the rescue function and are certain that he can help them with whatever hurts them.

6.   The Administrator:

The administrator sets the "tone" for any nursing home. Generally an administrator is a 50 year old woman or man with a high school education. A few have additional training, such as degrees in physical therapy, nursing or any subject from archeology to music. In New York State, however, all must be certified in "Geriatrics" by attending 100 clock hours of lectures on that subject.

There is one factor which all of these caretakers have in common: they have entered the field of nursing home administration to earn a generally good livelihood with relatively little formal education for such an important position. In addition, they desire power. Power is what they have, since most of their employees are unskilled or semi-skilled workers like nurses aides, office clerks, laundry people, etc. Since the patients are often helpless the administrator wields this power not only over the employees but also over the residents of the nursing home. Nowhere else would a former bookkeeper, now administrator, be able to make life and death decisions. These decisions are given him through his ability to hire employees and make all decisions concerning the patients' care.

It is rare that the administrator mingles with the patients and when he does so it is only at the time of an "Open House," or to take "VIP's" through the facility.

The administrator is aggressive, domineering and guards his position with jealousy. If he is not the owner-operator he does not allow anyone near the proprietor for fear that his own position may be jeopardized by a subordinate's possible relationship with the owner.

The administrator is generally a very thrifty individual, running a tight budget, attempting to show as much profit as possible in order to keep his position and show his nursing home in a favorable light to investors.

Administrators have been known to visit the homes of patients or their bank safes together with the patient in order to help themselves to whatever they wanted "since they owe it to the nursing home anyway." When everything the patient has has been depleted and absorbed by the nursing home by such administrative tactics, the patients are then transferred to a dormitory type room to make way for "a private pay" patient. The wants and needs of the destitute aged patient are then ignored and he is called "greedy" and self seeking if he demands his possessions. Administrators are very thoughtful to familes of patients and cater to them with finesse.

7. The Aide:

The nurses aide is the most useful, most necessary and perhaps the hardest working of all nursing home staff. She has the opportunity for close relationships and therefore most often does have the closest relationships with the patients. She feeds and bathes her charges, makes their beds, caters to their needs and listens to their complaints. If she is a good aide she cheers up her patients, knows the habits of their deceased parents, knows their unhappiness about their great niece Suzie who hasn't visited in a year, knows their likes and dislikes and sometimes even peels tomatoes or grapes for a patient who can't digest the skins. She has been known to bring in a slightly used pajama for a patient who is out of night-clothes, or a two ounce box of favorite chocolates to an especially loved total care patient.

The aide is grossly underpaid, often receiving merely the minimum wages paid in a particular region; has to clean up urine and feces; is in constant contact with helpless depressed people and if she were conscientious would need seventy-two hours in an eight hour shift. She is the recipient of the unhappiness of the patient, the nurse and all other personnel who feel upset about something in their immediate or not so immediate environment. The aide's job can be a very depressing one since death is always around her and she has the added responsibility of covering and/or wrapping the bodies of her charges after they have taken their last breath.

Because of the low status of the aide together with her low income, it does occur that she takes material things from patients, as well as food and other commodities from the nursing home which do not belong to her. There is also the aide who is so overwhelmed by misery and pressures that she disappears into the bathroom for extended periods of time, letting the patients' lights or buzzers go unnoticed. The night aide has the greatest opportunity for engaging in this kind of behavior since there is fewer personnel on the floor then, and therefore generally no one to "report" her. There is the occasional sadistic aide who handles patients in an unkind, physically rough manner. The patients are frail and riddled with medical problems in most cases so that the slightest movement is often painful. Thus, careless or unthinking pulling of the patient causes unbearable pain. For the most part, however, the aide is a caring individual who does the best she can in a difficult situation.

8.   The Nurse:

In a nursing home two kinds of nurses can be found - the registered nurse and the licensed practical nurse. The former has more education and hence more prestige and more latitude to make decisions. This description will concentrate on the R.N. She is the inexpensive physician of the nursing home. She is asked by both staff and patients to look at various physical problems of the patients, to diagnose, to treat with and without benefit of physician and to call for the doctor when she believes an absolute emergency has arisen. She has multitudinal responsibilities like distributing the daily medications at pre-scribed times, handling unusual feedings, those which do not take place through the oral cavity, administering oxygen when needed and filling out various forms. She sometimes has the responsibility to employ and supervise aides, orderlies, etc. Since the physician for the most part is unavailable and rarely seen around the nursing home, the patient turns for practical solutions and advice to the R.N. In the nursing home the nurse has more power and makes more decisions than in a hospital. She has almost no supervision, except from a peer, i.e., the directress of nurses, also a registered nurse. Therefore the treatment a patient receives is left to the degree of competence or incompetence of the nurse on a particular shift. Whenever the doctor does put in an appearance the nurse stands at absolute attention, holding the door for the doctor, pointing out the part of the body which she thinks needs examining and behaving like an automaton in the presence of the physician. Like the patient, she will quote the doctor frequently and appears to be obediently carrying out whatever orders he might have given.

9. The Social Worker:

The nursing home generally has two classes of "social workers:" a designee, an individual with limited education ranging anywhere from a high school diploma to a Bachelors degree in any subject, who works approximately forty hours per week, and a social work consultant. The main function of the designee is to fill out forms, to do paper work and to satisfy the state requirements. The required formats are meaningless pieces of paper which allegedly give the current socio-medical condition of the patient together with a recommendation for further disposition of the individual. Mostly they read, "Continued nursing home care is recommended since the patient needs assistance in Activities of Daily Living; is in need of skilled nursing care and has no one who is willing or able to take care of him outside of the institution." The designee has as many as 175 "patients" to service and therefore becomes discouraged and hardly has the opportunity to know the majority of inmates. Some designees have been known to be utilized as mail deliverers; purchasers of clothing (at night during non-working hours) and general scapegoats for angry administrators. Their function is very ill defined. In New York State it is spelled out in "The State Code of Social Services" but is not followed since the "social worker" has no power to carry out her prescribed function. If she complains too much she is dismissed. There are many untrained persons who would be able to fill out the "needed" papers in a manner similar to the designee already employed. Because of the lack of skill needed and the lack of caring on the part of nursing home administrators, the above condition exists.

The social work consultant spends about eight hours per month in the nursing home. During this time she talks with the designee about the general frustrations of the job and together they "plot" to create a better atmosphere for the patient and a more tenable situation for the designee. Since the consultant is an employee of the nursing home he cannot expose the deplorable conditions to higher authorities without jeopardizing his position. He would be summarily dismissed should he speak "the truth." Although it is one of the functions of the consultant to hold in-service training sessions he is rarely given the opportunity to do this and is generally excluded from the agenda. Any suggestions he might make to the administrator are tabled and involved in "the eternal waiting game."

The social worker of the State Department of Welfare appears at the nursing home several times a year. She can be a very experienced or a wholly inexperienced Masters degree social worker who definitely knows no more, if not less, than the consultant. She is full of good ideas and advice and chooses to question some minute detail concerning a case of the consultant and the designee. For instance, she will ask whether this particular nursing home is the best resource for a young total-care patient. When asked for suggestions she has no constructive ones - all nursing homes she mentions have already been tried and have rejected the patient. She will ask for reforms which the nursing home administrator will not grant under any circumstances. She has a conference with the administrator who later tells the designee that the representative from the State does not know what she is talking about or with whom. Thus the patient care does not improve, only the designee and the consultant become more anxious as their conflicts and feelings of frustration increase. The State's "watchdogs" accomplishments are zero.

PART IV

Staff Attitudes Toward Nursing Home Patients

In 1969, Larson, Knapp and Zuckerman[1] reminded us that "what trans-
pires in interpersonal communication is a function of the attitudes,
assumptions and sentiments which one person holds about another."[2] A
number of reports concerning nursing homes agree with them and the present authors and "testify to the importance of attitudes in the staff-
patient interaction."[3] Therefore we conducted an intensive investiga-
tion of such attitudes in two nursing homes, using the earlier work of
Larson, Knapp and Zuckerman as a model.

One of the nursing homes investigated is a public health related
facility located in a large dormitory on the campus of a state college.
As a branch of a larger county home and infirmary, this facility has no
separate administration, nor staff, but is administered and staffed by
the main home and infirmary located in a rural area, some twenty miles
distant. The home studied here houses 280 patients.

The second nursing home studied is a privately owned, profit making
venture. This facility is located in a suburb of a large city. In this
home both total nursing care and health related care are available on
the same premises. The administration and staff are present within the
facility which houses about 170 patients.

Following Larson, et al., a five factor interview schedule was prepared and a group of 53 employees in both nursing homes was asked to
evaluate a total of 28 questions arranged according to the significance
of each factor with reference to: (1) Rejection of Dissimilarities;
(2) Receptivity to Close Personal Relations; (3) Sorrow; (4) Service
Orientation, and (5) Rigid Expectations. Interviews were conducted by
trained professionals and by well prepared senior students. Staff members were asked to respond to each item on a scale of three possibilities, i.e., ranging from "agree" with the statement, to "disagree" and
"don't know." The following results were obtained from this study:

TABLE 1 - A

STAFF PERCEPTIONS OF THE
SOCIAL CHARACTERISTICS OF AGED PATIENTS

Factor 1	Agree		Disagree		Don't Know	
	No.	%	No.	%	No.	%
1. People in nursing homes are different from the people you find anywhere else.	16	30	36	68	1	2
2. Most nursing home patients are friendlier than other people.	16	30	35	66	2	4
3. Most patients try harder to be nice than people outside nursing homes.	19	36	30	57	4	7
4. Nursing home patients have contributed to society for many years and deserve to be taken care of now that they need help.	47	89	4	7	2	4
5. People in nursing homes don't know how to take care of themselves.	13	25	32	60	8	15
6. Many times older patients act like children.	42	79	9	17	6	4

Discussion:

Most evident are the high rates of agreement with statements 4 and 6. We conclude from this that the preponderance of staff see the old and sick patient as a dependent, who, like a child, deserves and needs care. However, this also implies that the adult individual, as a nursing home patient, loses his adult status-role and is relegated to that of an infant. The consequences of this status change, particularly the loss of the right to self determination, in turn bring about most of those problems described in other parts of this study. Unlike children, however, adult dependency is viewed as unacceptable as indicated by the majority responses to statement 5 which alleges that patients could take care of themselves if they wanted to do so. In our culture, therefore, physical disability is seen as unacceptable and is treated as if it were a deliberate and malicious act which the patient could control and change at will.

TABLE 1 - B

STAFF ATTITUDES CONCERNING SIMILARITIES AND DISSIMILARITIES OF PATIENTS AS COMPARED WITH THE GENERAL POPULATION

No. of Statements	0		1		2		3		4		5		6	
	No.	%	No.	%	No.	%	No.	%	No.	%	No.	%	No.	%
Number and Percent of all staff respondents	2		5	10	15	29	14	27	11	22	4	8	2	4

This table indicates that two respondents do not agree with any statement concerning factor 1. However, 14 respondents agree with three of these statements. A total of 61% of all respondents agree with three or more statements in factor 1, thus indicating that they do indeed view nursing home patients as differing from the general population.

TABLE 1 - C

PROFESSIONAL AND NON-PROFESSIONAL STAFF ATTITUDES CONCERNING FACTOR 1

No. of Statements	0		1		2		3		4		5		6	
	No.	%	No.	%	No.	%	No.	%	No.	%	No.	%	No.	%
Professionals	2		3	14	10	48	7	33	1	5				23
Non-Professionals	2		2	7	5	17	7	23	10	33	4	13	2	7	30

It is clearly visible that non-professional personnel view nursing home patients as dissimilar from other people with far greater frequency than is true of professional personnel. Thus, only 38% of the professionals but 76% of the non-professionals agree with three or more of the statements in factor 1.

67

TABLE 2 - A

STAFF PERCEPTIONS OF PATIENTS' EXPECTATIONS
CONCERNING STAFF BEHAVIOR

Factor 2	Agree No.	%	Disagree No.	%	Don't Know No.	%
1. Most patients expect you to get involved with them.	35	66	13	25	5	9
2. People who work in nursing homes have to spend more time with patients than they want to.	16	30	36	68	1	2
3. Most of the patients think that the staff is here only to wait on them.	27	51	23	43	3	6
4. Sometimes the patients get too attached to you.	42	79	11	21		
5. I don't believe in spoiling patients.	25	47	14	26	14	27
6. I especially like those patients who talk a lot about their own interests and hobbies.	25	47	25	47	3	6
7. People who work in nursing homes have to guard against getting too attached to the patients.	34	64	18	34	1	2
8. It is easy to get to know the patients real well.	30	57	18	34	5	9

Discussion:

Although the staff recognizes that the patients wish to be involved with them, the staff makes considerable effort to avoid this, since little reciprocity is expected. In part this is seen as dangerous because the age of the patients almost guarantees a short live relationship and the staff needs to protect itself against the ever present threat of death. Death of course means separation, loss and ultimate rejection.

This effort to remain uninvolved is also related to the staff's need to protect itself against constant demands for money, time and affection which the staff cannot dispense freely because of their own needs and lack of resources.

TABLE 2 - B

FACTOR 2

STAFF ATTITUDES CONCERNING CLOSE PERSONAL RELATIONS WITH PATIENTS

No. of Statements	0		1		2		3		4		5		6		7		8	
	No.	%	No.	%	No.	%	No.	%	No.	%	No.	%	No.	%	No.	%	No.	%
Number & Percent of all staff respondents			1		4	8	12	23	8	15	15	29	9	17	3	6	1	2

This table indicates that 92% of staff agree with three or more statements to the effect that close personal relations with patients are unacceptable.

TABLE 2 - C

PROFESSIONAL AND NON-PROFESSIONAL STAFF ATTITUDES CONCERNING FACTOR 2

No. of Statements	0		1		2		3		4		5		6		7		8		
	No.	%	No.	%	No.	%	No.	%	No.	%	No.	%	No.	%	No.	%	No.	%	
Professionals			1		3	14	4	18	4	18	6	27	5	23					86
Non-Professionals					1	3	8	27	4	13	9	30	4	14	3	10	1	3	97

No significant difference in attitudes between professional and non-professional staff exists in this area. Eighty-six percent of all professionals and 97% of all non-professionals agree with three or more statements revealing an unwillingness to enter into close personal relations with patients.

69

TABLE 3

STAFF PERCEPTION OF ATTITUDES, SENTIMENTS AND ASSUMPTIONS
WHICH ARE APPROPRIATE AND WHICH ARE INAPPROPRIATE FOR INDIVIDUALS
WORKING WITH AN AGED POPULATION

Factor 3	Agree		Disagree		Don't Know	
	No.	%	No.	%	No.	%
1. I feel sorry for the families of patients.	8	15	39	74	6	11
2. I don't think that I will ever let myself be placed in a nursing home.	16	30	15	28	22	42
3. People in nursing homes are "forgotten souls".	29	55	19	36	5	9
4. I really don't feel sorry for nursing home patients.	16	30	26	49	11	21
5. I am always amazed to find that nursing home patients enjoy life as much as they do.	31	58	20	38	2	4
6. I enjoy working in nursing homes because I realize that someday I will need someone to take care of me.	26	49	25	47	2	4

Discussion:

More than half of the staff readily agree that nursing home patients are "forgotten souls". Employees of nursing homes find it difficult to understand how a patient can enjoy life in those circumstances.

The staff is sympathetic to the condition of being a nursing home patient and identifies enough to want to avoid becoming a patient themselves. Staff give to themselves by giving to the patients and thereby feel that they can avoid the need to become a patient themselves.

This is almost as if the position of nursing home staff wards off the evil spirits.

TABLE 3 – A

FACTOR 3

STAFF ATTITUDES REPRESENTING SYMPATHY FOR PATIENTS AND THEIR FAMILIES

No. of Statements	0		1		2		3		4		5		6	
	No.	%	No.	%	No.	%	No.	%	No.	%	No.	%	No.	%
Number and Percent of all staff respondents	10	19	10	19			15	28	12	23	5	9	1	2

This table indicates that 62% of respondents agree with three or more statements which view the nursing home patient as an object of sympathy.

TABLE 3 – B

PROFESSIONAL AND NON-PROFESSIONAL STAFF ATTITUDES CONCERNING FACTOR 3

No. of Statements	0		1		2		3		4		5		6	
	No.	%	No.	%	No.	%	No.	%	No.	%	No.	%	No.	%
Professionals	6	26	2	9			6	26	7	30	2	9		
Non-Professionals	4	13	8	27			9	30	5	17	3	10	1	3

No significant differences exist between professionals and non-professionals concerning the amount of sympathy for patients. Thus, 65% of professionals and 60% of non-professionals agree with three or more statements in this factor.

TABLE 4

STAFF DESCRIPTIONS OF AGED INDIVIDUALS
WHO ARE MOST "APPEALING" TO THE STAFF

Factor 4	Agree		Disagree		Don't Know	
	No.	%	No.	%	No.	%
1. Most patients would rather do things for themselves instead of having you do them.	28	53	16	30	9	17
2. Some patients think you will do whatever they want you to do.	45	85	4	7.5	4	7.5
3. I enjoy this kind of work because you see the same people day after day, and I like things to be stable.	18	34	34	60	3	6
4. It is my duty to see that the patients get what they need.	46	87	6	11	1	2

Discussion:

While the staff is philosophically in agreement with the view that it is their duty to meet the needs of the patients, they also recognize that many patients would rather do many things for themselves.

At the same time the staff feels overburdened by the expectations they believe the patients have of them.

Those divergent views and demands create conflict and frustration for the staff and the patients and become at least one source of the aggression which is directed toward the patient population.

TABLE 4 - A

FACTOR 4

STAFF ATTITUDES INDICATING A "SERVICE ORIENTATION"

	0		1		2		3		4	
No. of Statements	No.	%	No.	%	No.	%	No.	%	No.	%
Number and Percent of all staff respondents			4	8	15	28	28	53	6	11

This table indicates that 14% of respondents (staff) feel that patients are imposing on them and that they (the staff) prefer not to be disturbed. There is a strong feeling against a service orientation. This is exhibited by the degree of agreement with two or more statements on this factor.

TABLE 4 - B

PROFESSIONAL AND NON-PROFESSIONAL STAFF ATTITUDES CONCERNING FACTOR 4

	0		1		2		3		4	
No. of Statements	No.	%	No.	%	No.	%	No.	%	No.	%
Professionals					8	35	13	56	2	9
Non-Professionals			4	13	7	23	15	50	4	13

While all professional staff agrees with two or more statements, only 87% of non-professionals have this view.

73

TABLE 5

STAFF PERCEPTIONS OF AGED INDIVIDUALS
WHO ARE LEAST "APPEALING" TO THE STAFF

Factor 5	Agree No.	%	Disagree No.	%	Don't Know No.	%
1. Most of the patients have set ideas and are pretty stubborn about most things.	33	63	14	27	5	10
2. The most attractive thing about a job in the nursing home is the pay.	3	6	49	94		
3. Most patients are not thankful for what they have.	14	26	26	49	13	25
4. The only patients I like are the ones that are happy, cheerful and friendly.	2	4	50	94	1	2

Discussion:

While the staff recognize a certain amount of self direction by the patients, this is called "stubborness" and is attributed to "set ideas". The same trait in younger adults is of course praised as determination and strength. However, since nursing home patient are viewed as children, this attribute is interpreted unfavorably and becomes a source o annoyance.

While many staff are intellectually able to recognize that they should like everyone equally, not only those who appear "happy, cheerful and friendly," they nevertheless fin patient resistance very difficult to handle because such resistance prevents the fulfill ment of institutional routines. Staff members often fear that they will be blamed for not carrying out policies and procedures which patients resist.

It is also significant that almost all staff feel underpaid and are not serving in the nursing home for the salary. Wages are seen as very unattractive. As a result there is a large turnover in nursing home staff.

TABLE 5 - A

FACTOR 5

STAFF ATTITUDE CONCERNING THE "PROPER BEHAVIOR" OF PATIENTS

	No. of Statements	0		1		2		3		4	
		No.	%	No.	%	No.	%	No.	%	No.	%
Number and Percent of all staff respondents	36	15	88	2	12						

More than two-thirds of all respondents disagree with all of the statements on this factor. Only a few agree with one or two statements and nobody will agree with three or four of them. This indicates that staff do not expect "proper" behavior from patients.

TABLE 5 - B

PROFESSIONAL AND NON-PROFESSIONAL STAFF ATTITUDES CONCERNING FACTOR 5

	No. of Statements	0		1		2		3		4	
		No.	%	No.	%	No.	%	No.	%	No.	%
Professionals	18	4	80	1	20						
Non-Professionals	18	11	92	1	8						

No significant difference exists between professional and non-professional responses to this factor.

PART V

Recommendations

Nursing homes at their best are not ideal places for the elderly. It is recognized however that there are individuals who have little choice and must reside within these facilities. It has been recognized that being placed into a nursing home connotes death for many patients and they know that the only way that they will leave the premises of the Home will be in a pine box. In order to enable the patient to live more comfortably during his stay in a convalescent facility the following recommendations are made:

1. Screening of staff before they are hired - culling out the problematic employees who are grossly character disordered. This can be done through interviewing techniques, references and observation.

2. Deleting of staff within the first three months or less who show strong sadistic tendencies, are crassly negligent and who show blatant lack of caring for their charges.

3. In-service training sessions for staff at frequent intervals. Treating all staff as an integral part of the treatment team, thus letting them know how important each is to the welfare of the patient.

4. Respecting the rights and dignities of the individual patient. For example, patients should be encouraged to sign their own

Social Security checks rather than having them arbitrarily
signed by the nursing home administration.

5. Nursing homes should be within easy distance of the patient's
    former home and familiar surroundings. The patient should not
    be placed very far away from the place where he lived, thus
    causing a greater feeling of segregation and isolation.

6. More utilization of the patient's family. Outreach by a social
    worker to the family of the patient to show them the need for
    visiting and doing things for the patient's welfare.

7. A full-time social worker should be employed who would work as
    an advocate for the patients. The worker would be employed by a
    "watch dog agency." The nursing home would have to reimburse
    the agency for this employee, but the nursing home would have no
    right to employ or discharge this employee.

8. Moving the patient out of the nursing home, back into the commu-
    nity whenever he is physically and emotionally ready to reenter
    the non-institutional milieu. This concept incorporates the
    readying of the individual for this step almost as soon as he
    enters the nursing home. The same must be done with the family
    of the patient - whenever there is family.

9. The patient should be given an opportunity to earn spending money
    selling items in an institutional store. If somehow feasible the
    potential patient should be kept in the community in his own home
    with appropriate resources available. For example: the mobile

physician's unit which would meet medical emergencies almost
instantly at a minimal cost to the individual; community day
care centers available so that the potential patient would
have a stimulating outlet during the day and be returned to
his home or his family's home at night. Transportation at a
minimal cost should be made available from door to door for
the person who is unable to wait for public transportation
because of health or other reasons; more senior citizen housing near shopping centers within walkable distance; community
kitchens within the housing unit should be made available
with one or several staff members on duty around the clock
should a person need help. The staff member could be a homemaker who would parcel out her time to each separate housing
unit, thus helping the incapacitated person with household
duties, baths or other activities of daily living.

There are many more possibilities within the realms of reality in
helping potential nursing home patients keep their dignity and enable them
to live more successfully within the human family.

APPENDIX

THE RIGHTS OF PATIENTS

by Robert Bainum

Administrator of Fairfax Nursing Home
Fairfax, Virginia

An elderly patient came up to a nursing home receptionist and requested her to mail some cards for him. "Leave the cards here," the receptionist replied, "and I will read them and then decide if I should mail them or not." To me this was a violation of this man's rights. True, he may write some "screwball" letters or cards, but this is his right and that right was violated.

The other day I was talking with a lady who directs a county health department program regulating nursing homes. She said that one of the problems that her office faced was seeing that patients received their mail!

Hundreds of patients have their mail censored unnecessarily, and their telephone calls monitored, and even their visitors restricted when one relative does not want another to visit the patient. These are seemingly little things, perhaps, and may appear even more so because the patient is ill, but it must be remembered that life is made up of hundreds of little things. These little things are important, especially when they concern the rights of people.

In this country every person possesses rights. Some of these rights are called "inalienable rights," or rights that cannot be transferred or assigned to another. Yes, every patient in every nursing home still possesses these rights.

"But," you say, "if I let my patients enjoy these rights, they would hurt themselves, or they would cease to be patients - they would run off." No doubt there are some cases where the court must curtail an individual's rights, but unless the court has specifically done this, we as nursing home administrators are violating the law and the person's human rights if we deny them any of the following:

The right to be the master of his own destiny.

The right to choose his own doctor.

The right to discharge the doctor.

The right to refuse medication or treatment.

The right to understand his illness and to be fully informed as to the nature, treatment and the medication for it.

The right to have everything in the nursing home program designed for his health, prevention of disease and accident.

The right to be restrained only when it is in strict accordance with the doctor's orders and the law.

The right of his medical treatment and personal problems to be kept in confidence.

The right to wear his own clothes and be dressed daily. (Nakedness has been a sign of guilt and indecency since Adam and Eve.)

The right to choose whom he will or will not live with.

The right to leave the nursing home at any time.

The right to legal counsel at any time that he requests.

The right, as a member of family, to receive information about members of his family or friends, whether good or bad, joyful or sorrowful.

The right to have visitors, such as friends and relatives, as long as he chooses to receive them.

The right to be counted as curable.

The right to live a full life and to make plans for the future.

The right to privacy in his communication, such as using the telephone and receiving and mailing letters.

The right to be religious or not to be religious.

The right to his personal property and his money.

The right to be treated as alive until pronounced dead by a licensed physician.

The right to have his orders followed concerning the burial of his remains at the time of his death.

When a patient comes to the point physically or mentally where it would be dangerous for him to exercise these rights, the patient's attorney or family should go to court and have the person declared incompetent. Then the rights that the patient possessed put into the custody of a person appointed by the court.

Of all the books that have been written about hospitals, doctors, nurses, medical personnel and nursing homes, I could find only two books in the Library of Congress that mentioned the subject about the rights of a patient. In 1959 the National League of Nursing at a convention adopted the following "Patient's Bill of Rights."

"1. To receive the nursing care necessary to help him regain or maintain his maximum degree of health."

"2. To have personnel care for him that are qualified through education, experience, and personality, to carry out the services for which they are responsible."

"3. To have nursing personnel caring for him that will be sensitive to his feelings and responsive to his needs."

"4. Within limits determined by the doctor, to teach the patient and his family about his illness so that the patient can help himself, and his family can understand and help him."

"5. To have plans made with him and his family...so that, if possible, continuing nursing and other necessary services will be available to him throughout the period of his need."

"6. For nursing personnel to assist in keeping adequate records and treat with confidence all personal matters that relate to the patient."

"7. For efforts to be made by nursing personnel to adjust surroundings of the patient so as to help him maintain or recover his health."

Every patient in a nursing home is a person and every person is made up of himself and his family. Yes, no person is complete without his family, or no family is complete without one of its members. Therefore, when a member of a family becomes a patient in a nursing home, this gravely affects the rest of the members of the family. The family is concerned over the patient's care, suffering, his future and his chances of getting well. He faces the problem of finances, and the social problems that come along from having a person taken from his home, such as loneliness. There is the problem of visiting the patient, the feelings of guilt, and many other things that seem to frustrate the family. Thus it can be seen that each member of the family has an interest in the patient and his stay in the nursing home. Because of this, every nursing home has an obligation to every member of the family and even to the friends of the patient. The family has the right to expect the following from the nursing home and the staff:

1. That every phase of treatment, medication and care will be done in an efficient way under a physician's orders.

2. That all the rights of the patient will be protected and honored.

3. That the home will keep them promptly informed of the patient's health.

4. That they will be given a full explanation regarding the nature of the patient's illness, so that they may judge the effectiveness of the overall care program.

5. That they may expect the nursing home to do everything possible to increase the health and well-being of the patient.

6. That the nursing home will follow the doctor's orders regarding medical treatment and not those of the relatives.

7. That they have a right to be permitted to visit the patient.

8. That no one member of the family is to decide who may or may not see their loved one.

9. That no nurse or other personnel is to alienate the patient's affections.

10. That the staff of the nursing home will not take sides in family arguments.

11. That they have the right to be notified and to be with the patient when he is dying.

12. That the expenses, charges, and basic services will not be charged before the family is notified.

13. That the patient's money and personal property will be given only to the representative of the estate upon his death.

An article in the February 3, 1953, issue of Look magazine sums up the rights of a patient: (Although written for hospitals, it applies equally to nursing homes.)

"In the official report written by the investigators from the California Medical Assn., one section discusses what changes in hospital routine must be made to satisfy the emotional needs of patients. Here, in their own words, is how investigators spell out the basic rights of patients:

"Hospitals should be so arranged as to maintain in a patient everything that is health - his desire to save face, to maintain identity, to remain as active as his physical condition permits. At present, our hospitals tend to destroy in the patient any attempt at self-determination and actually cause him to become emotionally, if not physically, sicker than he was when he entered the hospital.

"Being clothed, rather than draped in a muslin bag, is not only a symbol of dignity, but a symbol of social importance, and hence contributes to a person's maintenance of self-image and a willingness to get better and assume his social obligations. Therefore, upon entering a hospital, the decision about immediately disrobing and going to bed should be based on a consideration of bed rest. If and when a patient disrobes, he should be able to keep his clothes in a nearby locker or closet, or to have available suitable dress in order to be clothed whenever possible. If bed clothes are essential, the patient should use his own...."

"A patient should be permitted to retain his personal belongings and whatever money or property he believes he needs, without a staff member fingering through them as if the staff were now the patient's guardian."

"The autonomy of the patient should be maintained as much as possible. He should be informed about his progress, and about the exact state of his temperature, blood pressure, etc., unless such information is contraindicated by a patient's mental condition. If possible, he should be asked to chart his own temperature, weight, etc., and thereby be permitted to take an active part in his own therapy."

"Hours for waking, washing, eating and going to sleep should be flexi-

ble; a patient's schedule should not be determined only by the convenience of the nurses' work shift. Flexibility at mealtime, for example,
allowing a leeway of one to two hours within which patients may choose
to take their meals, would certainly be possible, if the wards were
organized accordingly. Sleeping hours should approximate sleeping time
of adults on the outside rather than the bedtime of small children."

We must remember that no patient is an island to himself. That
is, life is intertwined with other members of his family. He will not
be satisfied or complete unless his family can be assured that he is
getting the care, comfort and love that he should have.

In nursing home circles it has always been said that you do not
have trouble with the patients - you have it with their families. If
the rights of the patients and the families are more closely guarded
and honored by the nursing home, I am sure that we would have less trouble with the families.

I believe that the rights of the patients in the nursing home is
one of the biggest challenges facing the nursing home profession at this
time. I believe that the rights of many patients are being violated,
especially in the field of considering the patient as a person and
understanding that he still possesses all the rights of another citizen.

Mrs. Minna Fields, in a book called Patients are People, says that a
most important part of the treatment of a patient is the appreciation of
the dignity of the individual and the respect for his rights as a human
being, regardless of the stage of his illness or the degree of his impair-
ment.

NOTES

PART I

1. Burger, Robert E., "Commercializing the Aged," in *Annual Editions: Readings in Social Problems* 1973/1974, Guilford, Conn., The Dushkin Publishing Group, 1973, pp. 207-209.

2. *Statistical Abstracts of the U.S., 93rd Annual Edition*, United States Department of Commerce, United States Bureau of the Census, 1972, p. 31.

3. Birren, James E., "The Abuse of the Urban Aged," in *Change: Readings in Sociology and Human Behavior*, Del Mar, Cal., Communications Research Machines, Inc., 1972, pp. 94-96.

4. Caplowitz, David, *The Poor Pay More*, N.Y., The Free Press, 1968.

5. Statistical Abstracts, *op.cit.*, p. 31.

6. Burger, *op.cit.*, p. 208.

7. Berg, R. S., Browning, F. E., Hill, J. G. and Wenkert, W., "Assessing the Health Care Needs of the Aged," *Health Services Research*, Spring 1970, pp. 36-59.

8. Burger, *op.cit.*, p. 208.

9. Bunzel, Joseph H., "Recognition, Relevance and Deactivation of Gerontophobia: Theoretical Essay," *The Journal of the American Geriatrics Society*, Vol. XXI, No. 2, February 1973, pp. 73-80.

10. Congress of the U.S., Public Law 92-603, Sec. 265, October 1972.

11. Kosberg, Jordan I., "The Nursing Home: A Social Work Paradox," *Social Work*, Vol. 18, No. 2, March 1973, p. 105.

12. Rusalem, H. and Speiser, G., "The Meaningfulness of Work," *The Vocational Guidance Quarterly*, Vol. 12, Winter, 1963-64, pp. 119-122.

13. Ahrendt, Hannah, <u>Eichmann in Jerusalem</u>, The Viking Press, N.Y., 1963, p. 250.

14. Slocum, Walter, <u>Occupational Careers</u>, Chicago, Aldine Publishing, 1966, p. 76.

15. Hodge, Robert W., Seigel, Paul M. and Rossi, Peter H., "Occupational Prestige in the United States, 1925-1963," <u>American Journal of Sociology</u>, 70, November, 1964, pp. 286-302.

16. Mergers, Richard, "Childrens Rights, Normalization and Organizational Patterns of Institutions," <u>The Peabody Journal of Education</u>, Vol. 50, January 1973, pp. 128-134.

PART III

1. Bunzel, Joseph H., "Concept, Meaning and Treatment of Gerontophobia," <u>Zeitschrift fur Alternsferschung</u>, Band 25, Heft 1, January, 1971, pp. 15-18.

2. Bunzel, Joseph H., "Recognition, Relevance and Deactivation of Gerontophobia: Theoretical Essay," <u>The Journal of the American Geriatrics Society</u>, Vol. XXI, No. 2, February 1973, pp. 73-80.

3. Henigmann, John J., <u>The World of Man</u>, New York, Harper & Bros., 1959, p. 661.

4. Noss, John B., <u>Man's Religions</u>, New York, The MacMillan Co., 1956, p. 443.

PART IV

1. Larsen, Carl E., Knapp, Marl L. and Zuckerman, Isadore, "Staff-Resident Communication in Nursing Homes," <u>The Journal of Communication</u>, Vol. 19, December 1969, p. 308.

2. <u>Ibid</u>, p. 309.

3. <u>Ibid</u>, p. 309.